AIP DIET COOKBOOK FOR SENIORS

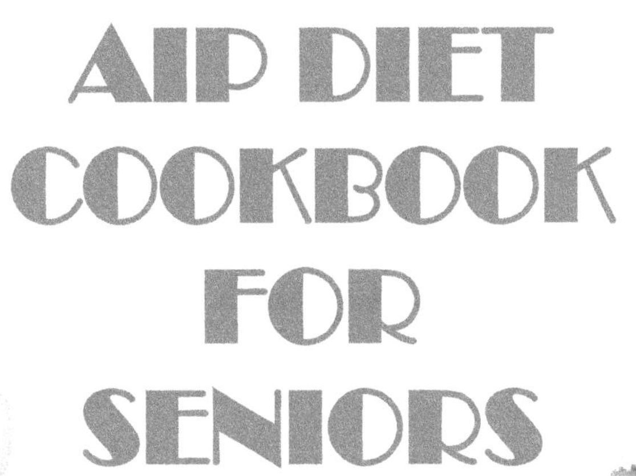

Dr. Kimberly Carlos

TABLE OF CONTENT

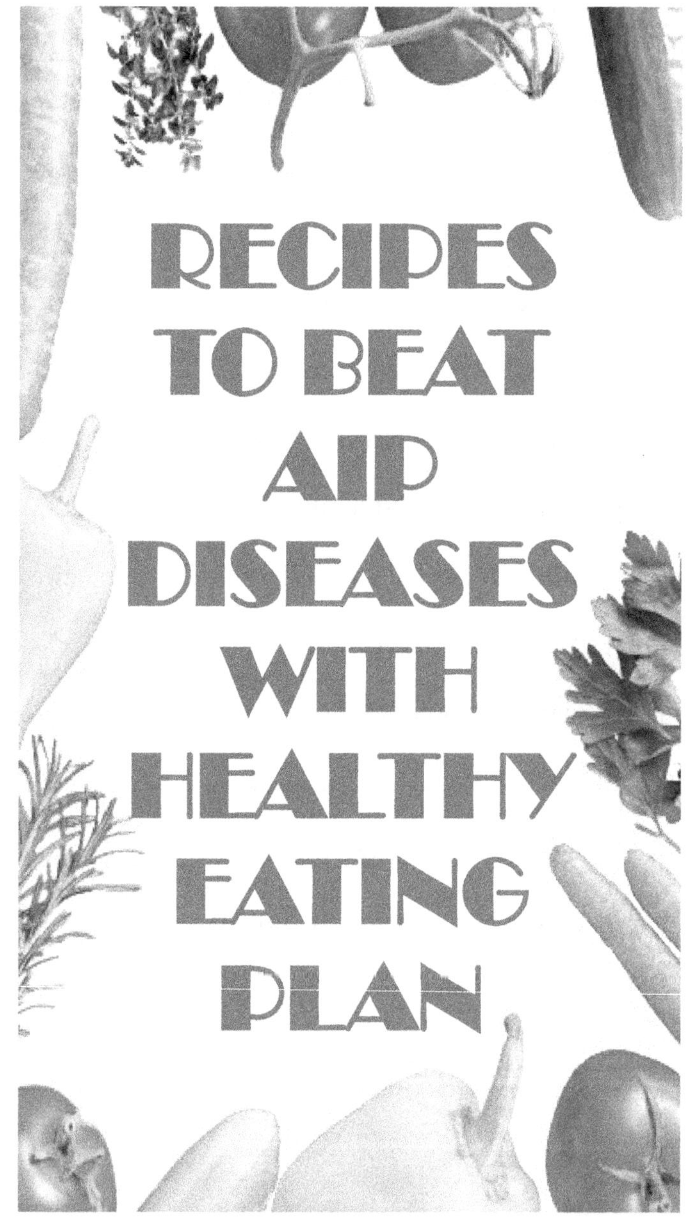

RECIPES TO BEAT AIP DISEASES WITH HEALTHY EATING PLAN

INTRODUCTION

In a world where health challenges seem to be on the rise, finding holistic and effective approaches to address autoimmune conditions has become paramount.

The Autoimmune Protocol (AIP) diet stands out as a transformative and science-backed solution, offering hope and healing to those grappling with autoimmune disorders.

Understanding Autoimmune Protocol (AIP):

Autoimmune diseases occur when the immune system mistakenly attacks healthy tissues, leading to chronic inflammation and a range of symptoms. AIP is a therapeutic diet specifically designed to alleviate these symptoms and promote healing by addressing the root causes of autoimmune conditions.

The Core Principles of AIP:

The AIP diet is built on the foundation of eliminating foods that may trigger inflammation and compromise gut health while emphasizing nutrient-dense, healing alternatives.

The core principles include:

1. Elimination Phase:

- Removal of common inflammatory foods: grains, dairy, legumes, nightshades, processed foods, and certain spices.

- Introduction of nutrient-rich foods: vegetables, fruits, lean proteins, and healthy fats.

2. Reintroduction Phase:

- Systematic reintroduction of eliminated foods to identify individual sensitivities.

- Personalization of the diet based on individual responses.

3. Focus on Gut Health:

- Emphasis on foods that support gut healing, such as bone broth, fermented foods, and collagen-rich sources.

- Recognition of the gut-immune system connection and its role in autoimmune conditions.

Adopting the AIP Diet:

Embarking on the AIP journey involves a thoughtful and gradual approach to allow the body to adjust to the new dietary guidelines.

Here's a step-by-step guide on how to adopt the AIP diet:

1. Educate Yourself:

- Gain a thorough understanding of AIP principles and its impact on autoimmune health.

- Read reputable resources, consult healthcare professionals, and connect with the AIP community for support.

2. Kitchen Detox:

- Clear your kitchen of eliminated foods to create an AIP-friendly environment.

- Stock up on AIP-approved ingredients, including a variety of vegetables, fruits, and high-quality proteins.

3. Meal Planning:

- Plan meals that align with AIP principles, incorporating a diverse range of nutrient-dense foods.

- Experiment with AIP recipes to discover delicious and satisfying alternatives.

4. Gradual Elimination:

- Gradually eliminate trigger foods rather than adopting the diet abruptly to minimize potential detox symptoms.

- Prioritize nutrient density to ensure you meet your nutritional needs during the elimination phase.

5. Seek Support:

- Connect with the AIP community for guidance, inspiration, and shared experiences.

- Consider working with a healthcare professional or a nutritionist familiar with AIP to tailor the diet to your specific needs.

6. Reintroduction and Personalization:

- Introduce eliminated foods one at a time during the reintroduction phase.

- Keep a food journal to track responses and identify potential sensitivities.

7. Lifestyle Factors:

- Embrace lifestyle changes that complement the AIP diet,

including stress management, quality sleep, and gentle exercise.

- Prioritize self-care to support overall well-being.

Scientific Basis and Efficacy:

Numerous scientific studies support the efficacy of the AIP diet in managing autoimmune conditions. The diet's focus on removing inflammatory triggers, supporting gut health, and addressing nutrient deficiencies aligns with current research on autoimmune disorders.

Challenges and Considerations:

While AIP offers immense potential for healing, it's essential to acknowledge the challenges associated with the diet. Social implications, potential nutrient deficiencies, and the need for personalized adjustments are factors that individuals may need to navigate.

The Autoimmune Protocol (AIP) diet stands as a beacon of hope for those seeking to manage and alleviate the symptoms of autoimmune disorders. By addressing the root causes of inflammation and prioritizing nutrient-dense, healing foods, individuals embarking on the AIP journey can experience a transformative shift toward better health and well-being.

The adoption of AIP involves a thoughtful and personalized approach, with the ultimate goal of empowering individuals to take control of their health and embrace a vibrant and balanced life.

As ongoing research continues to support the scientific basis of AIP, its potential to revolutionize autoimmune care remains a promising and exciting avenue for the future of holistic wellness.

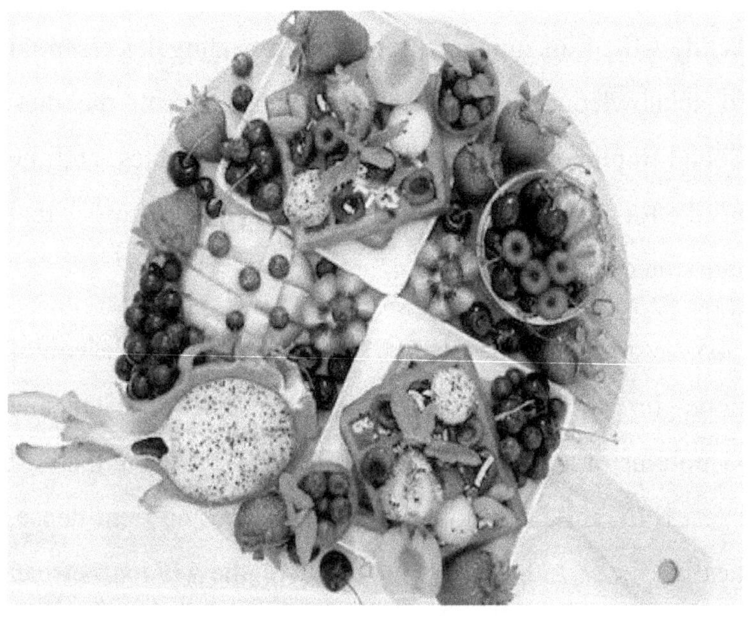

DELICIOUS AIP DIET RECIPES

1. AIP-Friendly Roasted Sweet Potato and Turkey Hash

Ingredients:

- 2 medium-sized sweet potatoes, peeled and diced

- 1 pound ground turkey

- 1 onion, finely chopped

- 2 cloves garlic, minced

- 1 teaspoon fresh rosemary, chopped

- 1 teaspoon fresh thyme, chopped

- Salt and pepper to taste

- 2 tablespoons coconut oil

Instructions:

1. Preheat your oven to 400°F (200°C).

2. Toss the diced sweet potatoes in 1 tablespoon of melted coconut oil and spread them on a baking sheet.

Roast for 20-25 minutes or until they are golden and tender.

3. In a large skillet, heat the remaining coconut oil over medium heat. Add the chopped onion and sauté until translucent.

4. Add the ground turkey to the skillet, breaking it apart with a spatula. Cook until browned.

5. Stir in the minced garlic, rosemary, thyme, salt, and pepper. Cook for an additional 2-3 minutes until the herbs are fragrant.

6. Add the roasted sweet potatoes to the skillet and mix everything together. Cook for another 5-7 minutes until the flavors meld.

7. Adjust the seasoning if necessary and serve warm.

2. AIP Coconut and Berry Chia Pudding

Ingredients:

- 1/4 cup chia seeds

- 1 cup coconut milk (full-fat, from a can)

- 1/2 teaspoon vanilla extract (make sure it's AIP-compliant)

- 1 tablespoon honey (optional)

- 1/2 cup mixed berries (blueberries, raspberries, strawberries)

Instructions:

1. In a bowl, combine the chia seeds, coconut milk, vanilla extract, and honey. Mix well.

2. Let the mixture sit for 5-10 minutes, stirring occasionally to prevent clumping.

3. Once the chia seeds have absorbed the liquid and the mixture has thickened, refrigerate it for at least 2 hours or overnight.

4. Before serving, stir the chia pudding to ensure an even consistency.

5. Spoon the chia pudding into serving bowls or glasses.

6. Top with mixed berries and serve chilled.

3. AIP-Friendly Zucchini Noodles with Avocado Pesto

Ingredients:

- 2 large zucchinis, spiralized

- 1 ripe avocado

- 1 cup fresh basil leaves

- 1/4 cup extra-virgin olive oil

- 1 clove garlic, minced

- Juice of 1 lemon

- Salt and pepper to taste

- Optional: nutritional yeast for a cheesy flavor

Instructions:

1. Spiralize the zucchinis into noodle-like strands.

2. In a blender or food processor, combine the avocado, basil, olive oil, minced garlic, lemon juice, salt, and pepper. Blend until you achieve a smooth, creamy consistency.

3. Toss the zucchini noodles with the avocado pesto until evenly coated.

4. Optional: Sprinkle nutritional yeast on top for a cheesy flavor.

5. Serve immediately and enjoy this refreshing and nutrient-packed dish.

4. AIP Baked Salmon with Lemon and Dill

Ingredients:

- 2 salmon fillets

- 2 tablespoons fresh dill, chopped

- 1 lemon, sliced

- 2 tablespoons avocado oil

- Salt and pepper to taste

Instructions:

1. Preheat your oven to 375°F (190°C).

2. Place the salmon fillets on a baking sheet lined with parchment paper.

3. Drizzle the avocado oil over the salmon fillets.

4. Sprinkle fresh dill, salt, and pepper evenly over the fillets.

5. Lay lemon slices on top of each fillet.

6. Bake in the preheated oven for 15-20 minutes or until the salmon flakes easily with a fork.

7. Remove from the oven, let it rest for a few minutes, and serve.

5. AIP Blueberry Coconut Flour Muffins

Ingredients:

- 1 cup coconut flour

- 1/2 cup coconut oil, melted

- 1/2 cup coconut milk

- 1/2 cup honey

- 4 large eggs

- 1 teaspoon vanilla extract (AIP-compliant)

- 1/2 teaspoon baking soda

- 1/4 teaspoon salt

- 1 cup fresh blueberries

Instructions:

1. Preheat your oven to 350°F (175°C) and line a muffin tin with paper liners.

2. In a bowl, whisk together the melted coconut oil, coconut milk, honey, eggs, and vanilla extract.

3. In a separate bowl, combine the coconut flour, baking soda, and salt.

4. Gradually add the dry ingredients to the wet ingredients, mixing until well combined.

5. Gently fold in the fresh blueberries.

6. Spoon the batter into the muffin cups, filling each about two-thirds full.

7. Bake for 20-25 minutes or until a toothpick inserted into the center comes out clean.

8. Allow the muffins to cool before serving.

6. AIP Turmeric Chicken Skillet

Ingredients:

- 2 boneless, skinless chicken breasts, sliced into strips

- 1 tablespoon coconut oil

- 1 teaspoon turmeric powder

- 1/2 teaspoon ground ginger

- 1/2 teaspoon garlic powder

- Salt and pepper to taste

- 1 cup broccoli florets

- 1 cup baby spinach

Instructions:

1. Heat coconut oil in a skillet over medium heat.

2. Season the chicken strips with turmeric, ginger, garlic powder, salt, and pepper.

3. Cook the chicken strips in the skillet until browned on all sides and fully cooked.

4. Add broccoli florets to the skillet and sauté until slightly tender.

5. Toss in baby spinach and cook until wilted.

6. Adjust seasoning if necessary and serve this vibrant and flavorful dish.

7. AIP Cucumber Avocado Salad

Ingredients:

- 2 cucumbers, thinly sliced

- 1 ripe avocado, diced

- 1/4 cup fresh cilantro, chopped

- 2 tablespoons extra-virgin olive oil

- Juice of 1 lime

- Salt and pepper to taste

Instructions:

1. In a bowl, combine the thinly sliced cucumbers, diced avocado, and chopped cilantro.

2. Drizzle extra-virgin olive oil over the salad.

3. Squeeze the lime juice over the ingredients.

4. Gently toss the salad until well combined.

5. Season with salt and pepper according to your taste.

6. Refrigerate for a short time to let the flavors meld before serving this refreshing and crisp AIP-friendly salad.

8. AIP Baked Sweet Potato Fries

Ingredients:

- 2 large sweet potatoes, peeled and cut into matchsticks

- 2 tablespoons coconut oil, melted

- 1 teaspoon dried rosemary

- 1/2 teaspoon sea salt

- 1/4 teaspoon garlic powder

Instructions:

1. Preheat the oven to 425°F (220°C).

2. In a bowl, toss sweet potato matchsticks with melted

coconut oil, rosemary, sea salt, and garlic powder until evenly coated.

3. Spread the sweet potatoes in a single layer on a baking sheet.

4. Bake for 25-30 minutes or until the fries are golden and crisp, flipping halfway through.

9. AIP Lemon Herb Grilled Chicken

Ingredients:

- 4 boneless, skinless chicken thighs

- Zest and juice of 1 lemon

- 2 tablespoons fresh parsley, chopped

- 1 tablespoon fresh oregano, chopped

- 2 cloves garlic, minced

- 2 tablespoons olive oil

- Salt and pepper to taste

Instructions:

1. In a bowl, mix lemon zest, lemon juice, chopped parsley, chopped oregano, minced garlic, olive oil, salt, and pepper to create a marinade.

2. Place the chicken thighs in the marinade, ensuring they are well coated. Marinate for at least 30 minutes.

3. Preheat the grill to medium-high heat.

4. Grill the chicken thighs for 6-8 minutes per side or until fully cooked and nicely charred.

10. AIP Berry Coconut Smoothie Bowl

Ingredients:

- 1 cup mixed berries (strawberries, blueberries, raspberries)

- 1 ripe banana

- 1/2 cup coconut milk

- 2 tablespoons shredded coconut

- A handful of fresh mint leaves (for garnish)

Instructions:

1. In a blender, combine mixed berries, banana, and coconut milk. Blend until smooth.

2. Pour the smoothie into a bowl.

3. Top with shredded coconut and garnish with fresh mint leaves.

4. Enjoy this nutrient-packed and visually appealing AIP-friendly smoothie bowl.

11. AIP Roasted Brussels Sprouts with Bacon

Ingredients:

- 1 pound Brussels sprouts, halved

- 4 slices AIP-compliant bacon, chopped

- 2 tablespoons olive oil

- 1 teaspoon garlic powder

- Salt and pepper to taste

Instructions:

1. Preheat the oven to 400°F (200°C).

2. In a large bowl, toss Brussels sprouts and chopped bacon with olive oil, garlic powder, salt, and pepper.

3. Spread the mixture on a baking sheet in a single layer.

4. Roast for 25-30 minutes or until the Brussels sprouts are crispy and golden.

12. AIP Grilled Pineapple Chicken Skewers

Ingredients:

- 1 pound chicken breast, cut into cubes

- 1 cup fresh pineapple chunks

- 2 tablespoons coconut aminos

- 1 tablespoon apple cider vinegar

- 1 teaspoon ground ginger

- 1 teaspoon garlic powder

- Salt and pepper to taste.

Instructions:

1. Preheat the grill to medium-high heat.

2. In a bowl, combine coconut aminos, apple cider vinegar, ground ginger, garlic powder, salt, and pepper to create a marinade.

3. Thread chicken cubes and pineapple chunks alternately onto skewers.

4. Brush the skewers with the marinade.

5. Grill for 10-12 minutes, turning occasionally, until the chicken is cooked through and has a nice char.

13. AIP Avocado Chocolate Pudding

Ingredients:

- 2 ripe avocados

- 1/4 cup carob powder

- 1/4 cup maple syrup

- 1/4 cup coconut milk

- 1 teaspoon vanilla extract

- Pinch of salt

Instructions:

1. Scoop the flesh of the avocados into a blender or food processor.

2. Add carob powder, maple syrup, coconut milk, vanilla extract, and a pinch of salt.

3. Blend until smooth and creamy.

4. Refrigerate for at least 30 minutes before serving.

14. AIP Zucchini Noodles with Pesto Sauce

Ingredients:

- 4 medium-sized zucchini, spiralized

- 1 cup fresh basil leaves

- 1/2 cup extra-virgin olive oil

- 1/4 cup pine nuts

- 2 cloves garlic

- Salt and pepper to taste

Instructions:

1. Spiralize the zucchini into noodles.

2. In a blender or food processor, combine basil, pine nuts, garlic, salt, and pepper.

3. With the blender running, slowly add the olive oil until the pesto is smooth.

4. Toss the zucchini noodles with the pesto sauce until well-coated.

15. AIP Sweet Potato Hash

Ingredients:

- 2 medium sweet potatoes, peeled and grated

- 1 onion, finely chopped

- 2 tablespoons coconut oil

- 1 teaspoon dried thyme

- Salt and pepper to taste

Instructions:

1. In a skillet, heat coconut oil over medium heat.

2. Add chopped onions and sauté until translucent.

3. Add grated sweet potatoes, thyme, salt, and pepper.

4. Cook, stirring occasionally, until the sweet potatoes are golden and cooked through.

16. AIP Turmeric Cauliflower Rice

Ingredients:

- 1 head cauliflower, riced

- 2 tablespoons coconut oil

- 1 teaspoon turmeric powder

- 1/2 teaspoon ground cumin

- Salt and pepper to taste

Instructions:

1. In a large skillet, heat coconut oil over medium heat.

2. Add cauliflower rice and sauté for 5-7 minutes until

tender.

3. Stir in turmeric powder, ground cumin, salt, and pepper.

4. Cook for an additional 2-3 minutes, ensuring the flavors are well combined.

17. AIP Cucumber Avocado Salad

Ingredients:

- 2 cucumbers, sliced

- 1 avocado, diced

- 1/4 cup fresh cilantro, chopped

- 2 tablespoons olive oil

- 1 tablespoon apple cider vinegar

- Salt and pepper to taste

Instructions:

1. In a bowl, combine sliced cucumbers, diced avocado, and chopped cilantro.

2. Drizzle olive oil and apple cider vinegar over the salad.

3. Toss gently to coat, and season with salt and pepper.

18. AIP Baked Apples with Cinnamon

Ingredients:

- 4 apples, cored and halved

- 2 tablespoons coconut oil, melted

- 1 teaspoon ground cinnamon

- 1/4 cup unsweetened shredded coconut

Instructions:

1. Preheat the oven to 375°F (190°C).

2. Place apple halves on a baking sheet.

3. Mix melted coconut oil and ground cinnamon, then brush the mixture over the apples.

4. Bake for 20-25 minutes or until apples are tender.

5. Sprinkle shredded coconut on top before serving.

19. AIP Lemon Herb Grilled Chicken

Ingredients:

- 4 boneless, skinless chicken breasts

- 2 tablespoons olive oil

- 2 tablespoons fresh lemon juice

- 2 cloves garlic, minced

- 1 teaspoon dried thyme

- Salt and pepper to taste

Instructions:

1. In a bowl, whisk together olive oil, lemon juice, minced garlic, thyme, salt, and pepper.

2. Place chicken breasts in a shallow dish and pour the marinade over them.

3. Marinate for at least 30 minutes.

4. Grill chicken over medium heat until fully cooked, about 6-8 minutes per side.

20. AIP Berry Coconut Smoothie

Ingredients:

- 1 cup mixed berries (blueberries, strawberries, raspberries)

- 1 cup coconut milk

- 1 tablespoon honey (optional)

- Ice cubes

Instructions:

1. In a blender, combine mixed berries, coconut milk, honey (if using), and ice cubes.

2. Blend until smooth and creamy.

3. Pour into glasses and enjoy this refreshing AIP-friendly smoothie.

21. AIP Roasted Brussels Sprouts

Ingredients:

- 1 pound Brussels sprouts, trimmed and halved

- 2 tablespoons coconut oil, melted

- 1 teaspoon garlic powder

- Salt and pepper to taste

Instructions:

1. Preheat the oven to 400°F (200°C).

2. In a bowl, toss Brussels sprouts with melted coconut oil, garlic powder, salt, and pepper.

3. Spread them on a baking sheet in a single layer.

4. Roast for 20-25 minutes, stirring halfway, until Brussels sprouts are golden and crispy.

22. AIP Sweet Potato and Bacon Hash

Ingredients:

- 2 medium sweet potatoes, peeled and diced

- 4 slices AIP-compliant bacon, chopped

- 1 onion, finely chopped

- 2 cloves garlic, minced

- 1 teaspoon dried rosemary

- Salt and pepper to taste

- Fresh parsley, chopped (for garnish)

Instructions:

1. In a skillet, cook chopped bacon until crispy. Remove and set aside.

2. In the same skillet, add diced sweet potatoes, onion, and garlic. Sauté until sweet potatoes are golden brown and cooked through.

3. Stir in cooked bacon, dried rosemary, salt, and pepper.

4. Garnish with fresh parsley before serving.

23. AIP Avocado Lime Tuna Salad

Ingredients:

- 2 cans AIP-compliant tuna, drained

- 2 avocados, diced

- 1 cucumber, diced

- 1/4 cup fresh cilantro, chopped

- Juice of 2 limes

- Salt and pepper to taste

Instructions:

1. In a bowl, combine drained tuna, diced avocados, diced cucumber, and chopped cilantro.

2. Squeeze lime juice over the mixture and gently toss to combine.

3. Season with salt and pepper to taste.

4. Serve as a refreshing tuna salad, perfect for a light AIP-friendly meal.

24. AIP Baked Cinnamon Apples

Ingredients:

- 4 apples, cored and sliced

- 2 tablespoons coconut oil, melted

- 1 teaspoon ground cinnamon

- 1/4 teaspoon ground ginger

- 1/4 teaspoon ground cloves

- 1 tablespoon maple syrup (optional)

Instructions:

1. Preheat the oven to 375°F (190°C).

2. In a bowl, toss apple slices with melted coconut oil, ground cinnamon, ground ginger, ground cloves, and maple syrup (if using).

3. Spread the coated apple slices on a baking sheet.

4. Bake for 20-25 minutes or until apples are tender and slightly caramelized.

25. AIP Cauliflower Fried Rice

Ingredients:

- 1 medium cauliflower, grated

- 2 tablespoons coconut oil

- 1 onion, finely chopped

- 2 carrots, diced

- 2 cups shredded cabbage

- 2 cloves garlic, minced

- 2 tablespoons coconut aminos

- Salt and pepper to taste

- Fresh chives, chopped (for garnish)

Instructions:

1. In a food processor, pulse the cauliflower until it resembles rice.

2. In a large skillet, heat coconut oil and sauté chopped onion and garlic until softened.

3. Add grated cauliflower, diced carrots, and shredded cabbage to the skillet. Cook until vegetables are tender.

4. Stir in coconut aminos and season with salt and pepper.

5. Garnish with fresh chives before serving.

26. AIP Lemon Herb Roasted Chicken

Ingredients:

- 1 whole chicken (about 4 pounds)

- 2 tablespoons olive oil

- 1 lemon, sliced

- 3 cloves garlic, minced

- 1 tablespoon fresh rosemary, chopped

- 1 tablespoon fresh thyme, chopped

- Salt and pepper to taste

Instructions:

1. Preheat the oven to 375°F (190°C).

2. Rinse the chicken and pat it dry with paper towels.

3. In a small bowl, mix olive oil, minced garlic, chopped rosemary, chopped thyme, salt, and pepper.

4. Rub the herb mixture all over the chicken, including under the skin.

5. Place lemon slices inside the chicken cavity.

6. Roast in the oven for about 1 hour or until the internal temperature reaches 165°F (74°C).

27. AIP Blueberry Coconut Smoothie

Ingredients:

- 1 cup frozen blueberries

- 1 cup coconut milk (AIP compliant)

- 1 tablespoon shredded coconut

- 1 tablespoon AIP-friendly collagen powder

- 1 teaspoon honey (optional)

Instructions:

1. Blend frozen blueberries, coconut milk, shredded coconut, collagen powder, and honey (if using) until smooth.

2. Pour into a glass and enjoy this nutrient-packed AIP smoothie.

28. AIP Zucchini Noodles with Pesto

Ingredients:

- 4 medium zucchinis, spiralized

- 1 cup fresh basil leaves

- 1/4 cup pine nuts

- 1/4 cup nutritional yeast

- 2 cloves garlic

- 1/2 cup AIP-compliant olive oil

- Salt and pepper to taste

Instructions:

1. In a food processor, combine basil, pine nuts, nutritional yeast, and garlic. Pulse until finely chopped.

2. With the processor running, slowly pour in olive oil until the pesto is well combined.

3. Toss spiralized zucchini with the pesto and season with salt and pepper.

29. AIP Turmeric Ginger Carrot Soup

Ingredients:

- 4 cups carrots, chopped

- 1 onion, chopped

- 2 cloves garlic, minced

- 1 tablespoon fresh ginger, grated

- 1 teaspoon ground turmeric

- 4 cups AIP-compliant chicken or vegetable broth

- Salt and pepper to taste

- Fresh cilantro, chopped (for garnish)

Instructions:

1. In a large pot, sauté chopped onion, minced garlic, and grated ginger until fragrant.

2. Add chopped carrots, ground turmeric, and AIP-compliant broth. Bring to a boil and simmer until carrots are tender.

3. Use an immersion blender to blend the soup until smooth.

4. Season with salt and pepper and garnish with fresh cilantro before serving.

30. AIP Baked Salmon with Lemon Dill Sauce

Ingredients:

- 4 salmon fillets

- 2 tablespoons AIP-compliant olive oil

- 1 teaspoon dried dill

- 1 teaspoon garlic powder

- Salt and pepper to taste

- Lemon slices (for garnish)

Instructions:

1. Preheat the oven to 400°F (200°C).

2. Place salmon fillets on a baking sheet.

3. Drizzle olive oil over the fillets and sprinkle with dried dill, garlic powder, salt, and pepper.

4. Bake in the preheated oven for about 15-20 minutes or

until the salmon is cooked through.

5. Garnish with lemon slices before serving.

31. AIP Sweet Potato Hash Browns

Ingredients:

- 2 medium sweet potatoes, peeled and grated

- 1 onion, finely chopped

- 2 tablespoons coconut oil

- 1 teaspoon dried thyme

- Salt and pepper to taste

- Fresh parsley, chopped (for garnish)

Instructions:

1. In a large skillet, heat coconut oil over medium heat.

2. Add chopped onion and sauté until translucent.

3. Add grated sweet potatoes and cook until they are golden brown and crispy.

4. Season with dried thyme, salt, and pepper.

5. Garnish with fresh parsley before serving.

32. AIP Avocado Lime Chicken Salad

Ingredients:

- 2 cups cooked chicken, shredded

- 1 avocado, diced

- 1 cucumber, diced

- 1 cup cherry tomatoes, halved

- 2 tablespoons AIP-compliant olive oil

- Juice of 1 lime

- Fresh cilantro, chopped

- Salt and pepper to taste

Instructions:

1. In a large bowl, combine shredded chicken, diced avocado, diced cucumber, and cherry tomatoes.

2. Drizzle olive oil and lime juice over the salad.

3. Add chopped cilantro, salt, and pepper. Toss until well

combined.

33. AIP Cauliflower Fried Rice

Ingredients:

- 1 medium cauliflower, grated

- 2 tablespoons coconut oil

- 1 onion, finely chopped

- 2 carrots, diced

- 2 cups broccoli florets

- 2 cloves garlic, minced

- 2 tablespoons coconut aminos

- Salt and pepper to taste

- Green onions, sliced (for garnish)

Instructions:

1. In a food processor, pulse the cauliflower until it resembles rice grains.

2. In a large skillet, heat coconut oil over medium heat.

3. Add chopped onion and garlic, sauté until fragrant.

4. Add diced carrots, broccoli, and cauliflower rice to the skillet. Cook until vegetables are tender.

5. Stir in coconut aminos, salt, and pepper. Garnish with sliced green onions.

34. AIP Lemon Herb Roasted Chicken

Ingredients:

- 1 whole chicken (about 4-5 pounds)

- 2 tablespoons AIP-compliant olive oil

- Zest and juice of 1 lemon

- 1 teaspoon dried rosemary

- 1 teaspoon dried thyme

- Salt and pepper to taste

Instructions:

1. Preheat the oven to 375°F (190°C).

2. Rinse the chicken and pat it dry with paper towels.

3. In a small bowl, mix olive oil, lemon zest, lemon juice, dried rosemary, dried thyme, salt, and pepper.

4. Rub the chicken with the mixture, ensuring it's well coated.

5. Place the chicken in a roasting pan and roast for about 1.5 to 2 hours or until the internal temperature reaches 165°F (74°C).

35. AIP Berry Coconut Smoothie Bowl

Ingredients:

- 1 cup mixed berries (blueberries, strawberries, raspberries)

- 1 ripe banana

- 1/2 cup coconut milk (AIP-compliant)

- 1 tablespoon shredded coconut

- AIP-friendly toppings: sliced kiwi, chopped mint

Instructions:

1. In a blender, combine mixed berries, banana, and coconut milk. Blend until smooth.

2. Pour the smoothie into a bowl.

3. Top with shredded coconut, sliced kiwi, and chopped mint.

36. AIP Zucchini Noodles with Pesto

Ingredients:

- 4 medium zucchinis, spiralized

- 1 cup fresh basil leaves

- 1/2 cup AIP-compliant olive oil

- 1/4 cup pine nuts

- 1 clove garlic, minced

- Salt and pepper to taste

- Lemon juice (optional)

Instructions:

1. Spiralize the zucchinis into noodles.

2. In a food processor, combine basil, olive oil, pine nuts, minced garlic, salt, and pepper. Blend until smooth.

3. Toss the zucchini noodles with the pesto sauce. Add a squeeze of lemon juice if desired.

37. AIP Roasted Root Vegetables

Ingredients:

- 3 cups mixed root vegetables (carrots, sweet potatoes, beets), peeled and diced

- 2 tablespoons AIP-compliant fat (coconut oil, lard, or duck fat)

- 1 teaspoon dried thyme

- Salt and pepper to taste

- Fresh parsley, chopped (for garnish)

Instructions:

1. Preheat the oven to 400°F (200°C).

2. In a bowl, toss diced root vegetables with AIP-compliant fat, dried thyme, salt, and pepper.

3. Spread the vegetables on a baking sheet and roast for about 30-40 minutes or until golden brown.

4. Garnish with chopped fresh parsley before serving.

38. AIP Avocado Tuna Salad

Ingredients:

- 2 cans AIP-compliant tuna, drained

- 1 ripe avocado, diced

- 1 cucumber, diced

- 2 tablespoons AIP-friendly mayonnaise

- 1 tablespoon fresh lemon juice

- Salt and pepper to taste

- Mixed greens for serving

Instructions:

1. In a bowl, combine drained tuna, diced avocado, and cucumber.

2. In a separate small bowl, mix AIP-friendly mayonnaise and fresh lemon juice.

3. Pour the mayo-lemon mixture over the tuna and veggies.

Gently toss until well combined.

4. Season with salt and pepper to taste.

5. Serve the tuna salad on a bed of mixed greens.

39. AIP Sweet Potato Hash

Ingredients:

- 2 medium sweet potatoes, peeled and grated

- 1 onion, finely chopped

- 2 tablespoons AIP-compliant fat (coconut oil, lard, or duck fat)

- 1 teaspoon ground cinnamon

- Salt and pepper to taste

- Fresh parsley, chopped (for garnish)

Instructions:

1. In a large skillet, heat AIP-compliant fat over medium heat.

2. Add chopped onion and sauté until translucent.

3. Add grated sweet potatoes to the skillet. Cook until the sweet potatoes are golden brown and cooked through.

4. Sprinkle ground cinnamon, salt, and pepper over the sweet potatoes. Stir to combine.

5. Garnish with chopped fresh parsley before serving.

40. AIP Grilled Lemon Herb Salmon

Ingredients:

- 4 salmon fillets

- 2 tablespoons AIP-compliant olive oil

- Zest and juice of 1 lemon

- 1 teaspoon dried dill

- 1 teaspoon dried oregano

- Salt and pepper to taste

Instructions:

1. Preheat the grill to medium-high heat.

2. In a small bowl, mix AIP-compliant olive oil, lemon zest,

lemon juice, dried dill, dried oregano, salt, and pepper.

3. Brush the salmon fillets with the lemon herb mixture.

4. Grill the salmon for about 4-5 minutes per side or until it flakes easily with a fork.

41. AIP Chicken and Vegetable Stir-Fry

Ingredients:

- 1 pound chicken breast, thinly sliced

- 2 cups broccoli florets

- 1 bell pepper, thinly sliced

- 2 carrots, julienned

- 3 tablespoons coconut aminos

- 2 tablespoons AIP-compliant fat (coconut oil or olive oil)

- 1 teaspoon ground ginger

- 2 cloves garlic, minced

- Salt and pepper to taste

- Fresh cilantro for garnish

Instructions:

1. Heat AIP-compliant fat in a large skillet over medium-high heat.

2. Add sliced chicken and cook until browned and cooked through.

3. Add broccoli, bell pepper, and julienned carrots to the skillet. Stir-fry until vegetables are tender-crisp.

4. In a small bowl, mix coconut aminos, ground ginger, minced garlic, salt, and pepper.

5. Pour the sauce over the chicken and vegetables. Stir well to coat.

6. Garnish with fresh cilantro before serving.

42. AIP Pumpkin Soup

Ingredients:

- 2 cups pumpkin puree

- 1 can (13.5 oz) coconut milk

- 1 onion, chopped

- 2 cloves garlic, minced

- 1 teaspoon ground turmeric

- 1 teaspoon ground ginger

- 1 tablespoon AIP-compliant fat (coconut oil or olive oil)

- Salt and pepper to taste

- Fresh chives for garnish

Instructions:

1. In a large pot, heat AIP-compliant fat over medium heat. Add chopped onion and sauté until translucent.

2. Add minced garlic, ground turmeric, and ground ginger. Stir well.

3. Pour in the pumpkin puree and coconut milk. Stir to combine.

4. Bring the soup to a simmer. Season with salt and pepper to taste.

5. Simmer for 15-20 minutes, allowing the flavors to meld.

6. Garnish with fresh chives before serving.

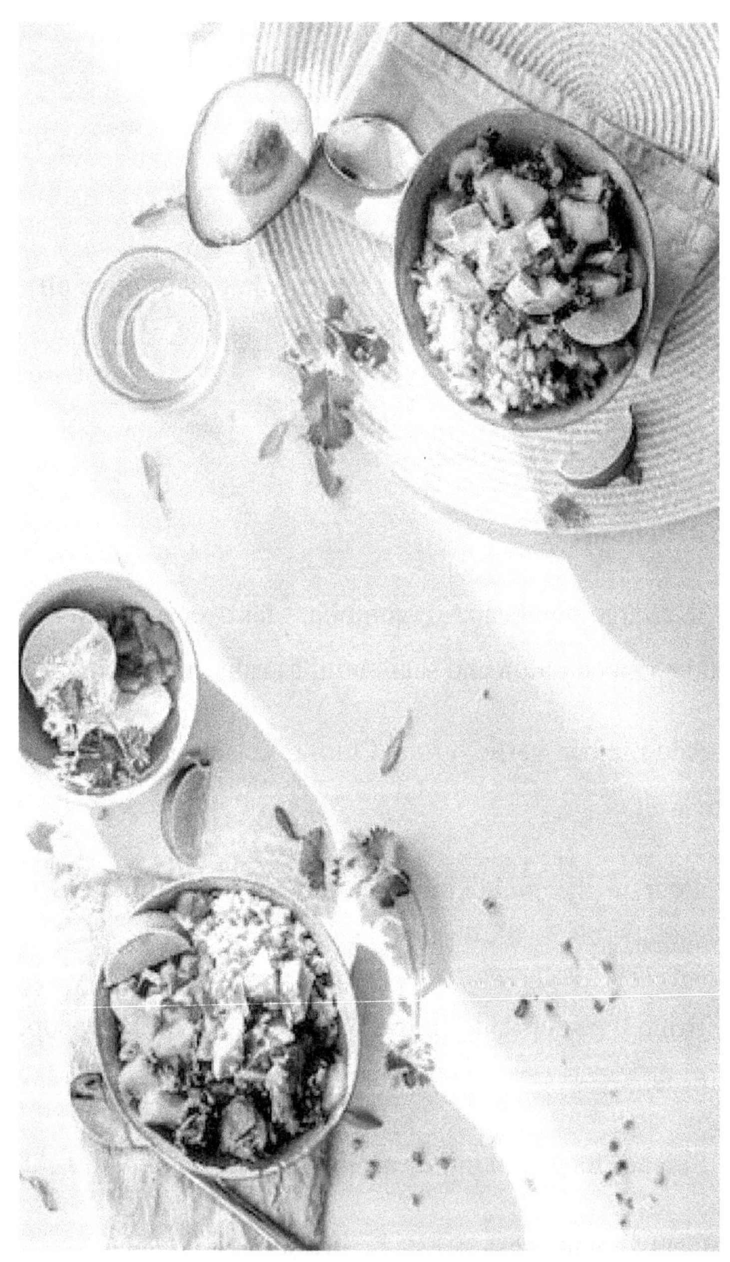

www.ingramcontent.com/pod-product-compliance
Lightning Source LLC
Chambersburg PA
CBHW061934270726
48660CB00007BA/2721